SUPER GUT HEALTH FOR WOMEN

Experience Healing, Effortless Weight Loss, Stress Liberation, Digestive Harmony, and Inflammation Soothing. Uncover Secrets to Your Best Self and Reclaim Joy in Every Moment!

DR. Maria Martin

Table of contents

Introduction

Unfortunately, health often takes a back place in today's fast-paced society. If you're looking for a wellness trend that has a comprehensive influence, one that jumps out is great gut health. Discover the deep meaning of "super gut health" and why it's crucial for women's overall wellness in this book.

The term "Super Gut Health" and its meaning

The lack of gastrointestinal problems is just one indicator of excellent gut health. Integral to this state of homeostasis is a diverse community of good bacteria, a strong intestinal lining, and efficient digestion. Achieving optimal gut health requires careful attention to this delicate equilibrium.

When the digestive system is in a condition of balance, it helps the body absorb nutrients, controls metabolism, and supports the immune system. This is the essence of great gut health. It is a proactive approach to general health, embracing the stomach as a vital participant in the complicated network of biological activities.

Importance of Gut Health for Women

For women, promoting gut health is not only about relieving stomach distress; it's about appreciating the essential role the gut plays in numerous facets of their health. From hormonal balance to mental well-being, the stomach functions as a keystone for overall health.

- **Hormonal Balance:** The gut microbiota regulates oestrogen metabolism, altering hormonal balance in women. A well-nourished gut helps to ease hormonal shifts during menstruation, pregnancy, and menopause.

- **Mental Well-being:** The gut-brain link is a fascinating element of gut health. The bidirectional link between the stomach and the brain regulates mood, stress levels, and cognitive performance. An unbalanced gut may lead to illnesses like anxiety and sadness.

- **Immune Support:** A substantial percentage of the immune system sits in the gut. A healthy gut with a diversified microbiome functions as a frontline defence against infections and boosts the body's capacity to fight off ailments.

Understanding the significance of gut health for women extends beyond treating particular health conditions; it becomes a proactive approach for boosting the overall quality of life.

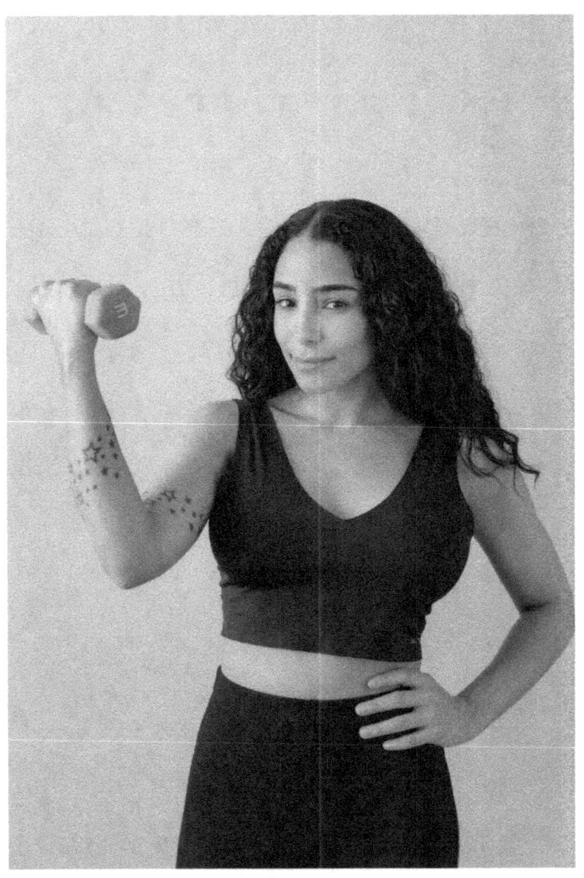

Chapter 1

The gut-brain connection.

Understanding the complex link between the stomach and the brain is an intriguing excursion into the heart of human physiology. This section delves into the complexity of the gut-brain link, including the gut-brain axis and its tremendous effect on mental health.

Investigating the Gut–Brain Axis

The gut-brain axis is a two-way communication mechanism that links the central nervous system to the enteric neural system in the gastrointestinal tract. This axis allows continuous communication between the stomach and the brain, which influences a variety of physiological and psychological activities.

- **Enteric Nervous System (ENS):** Also known as the "second brain," the enteric nervous system is a complex network of neurons implanted in the stomach lining. It acts autonomously but communicates with the central nervous system, where it plays an important role in digestion and gut health.

The vagus nerve is a significant conduit for communication between the gut and the brain. It sends messages in both ways, enabling the brain to impact gut function and vice versa. This ongoing discussion affects not just digestive functions, but also mental and emotional well-being.

- **Microbiome Influence:** The gut is home to billions of bacteria known collectively as the microbiome. This complex ecosystem of bacteria, viruses, and fungus interacts with the gut-brain axis to influence neurotransmitter synthesis and signalling.

Effects on Mental Health

Bidirectional communication along the gut-brain axis has significant consequences for mental health. The gut's status may impact mood, cognitive function, and even vulnerability to mental health issues.

The gut generates a variety of neurotransmitters, including serotonin, dopamine, and gamma-aminobutyric acid (GABA). The stomach produces the majority of serotonin, which is often related with mood control. An unbalanced stomach might affect neurotransmitter levels, perhaps leading to mood problems.

- **Stress reaction:** The stomach is crucial to the body's stress reaction. Chronic stress may disturb the equilibrium of the gut microbiota, resulting in inflammation and a weakened gut lining. This, in turn, may send messages to the brain, heightening tension and anxiety.

- **Inflammation and Mental Health:** Inflammatory processes in the stomach may cause systemic inflammation, which can damage the brain and contribute to mental health issues. According to research, there is a correlation between intestinal inflammation and disorders such as depression and anxiety.

- **Gut microbiota Diversity:** Maintaining a varied and healthy gut microbiota is critical for mental health. Dysbiosis, or a microbiome imbalance, has been linked to depression and neurodevelopmental abnormalities.

Memory and focus are examples of cognitive processes influenced by the gut-brain axis. A healthy stomach promotes adequate nutrition absorption, supplying vital nutrients for brain development.

Understanding the gut-brain connection's influence on mental health emphasises the need of maintaining a healthy gut for a robust and balanced mind.

Promoting the Gut-Brain Connection for Mental Health

Now that we've covered the complexity of the gut-brain connection, let's look at how to nourish this axis for maximum mental health.

• **Probiotics and Prebiotics:** Add probiotic-rich foods like yoghourt, kefir, and fermented vegetables to your daily diet. These meals bring helpful bacteria into the stomach, creating a healthy microbiome. Consume prebiotic-rich foods like garlic, onions, and bananas to help these beneficial microorganisms thrive.

• **Fiber-Rich Diet:** Fibre-rich foods promote regular bowel movements and feed healthy gut flora, boosting overall gut health. Whole grains, fruits, and vegetables are high in fibre.

• **Mindful Eating:** Enhance your gut-brain connection via mindful eating. Chew meals carefully, relishing each mouthful, and pay attention to your body's hunger and fullness signals. Mindful eating improves digestion and nutrition absorption.

- **Hydrate:** A healthy stomach requires enough fluids. Water maintains the mucosal membrane of the intestines and promotes overall digestive health. Aim to consume an appropriate quantity of water throughout the day.

- **Stress Management:** Add stress-reduction strategies like meditation, deep breathing, or yoga to your regimen. Managing stress has a good influence on the gut-brain axis, avoiding chronic stress from negatively affecting gut health.

- **Exercise:** Regular physical exercise promotes intestinal health. Exercise helps to maintain a varied gut flora and regulates the gut-brain axis. For total health, combine aerobic activity with strength training.

- **Quality sleep:** Prioritise quality sleep to maintain a healthy gut-brain connection. Sleep deprivation may upset the balance of gut flora and lead to increased stress.

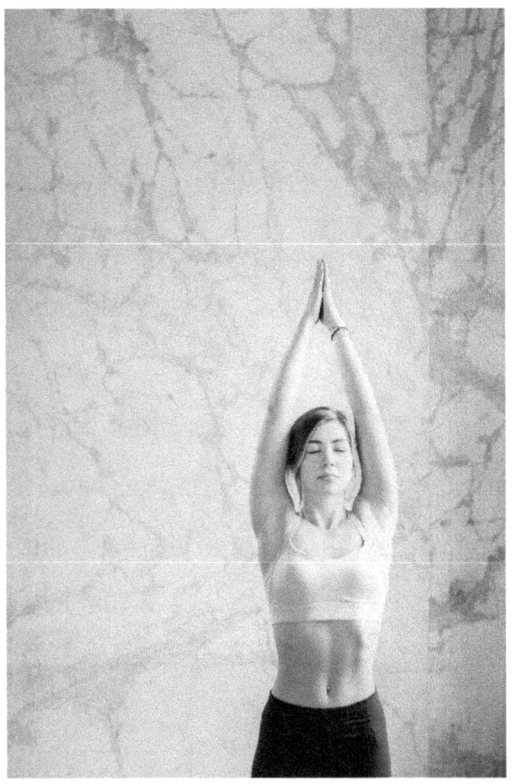

Chapter 2

Developing Ultimate Gut Health

Setting off on a path to achieve optimal gut health requires a deliberate fusion of mindful eating, a holistic perspective on health, and dietary modifications. The foundations of attaining optimal gut health will be discussed in this section, with particular attention paid to probiotics, food recommendations, and the role that water plays in supporting a healthy gut ecology.

Dietary Advice and Nutrition

- **Adopt a Wide Range of Diets:**

Maintaining a vibrant and varied diet is essential for a healthy gut microbiota. Include a variety of whole grains, legumes, fruits, and veggies. Your body and the billions of microbes in your stomach are both nourished by the distinct nutrients that each food category provides.

- **Make Fiber-Rich Foods a Priority:** Gut health is mostly dependent on fibre. It encourages regular bowel movements, fosters the development of advantageous microorganisms, and supports the preservation of the integrity of the gut lining. Make sure your daily meals include a good amount of fibre-rich foods such as whole grains, beans, nuts, seeds, and a range of fruits and vegetables.

- **Add prebiotics:** Prebiotics are indigestible fibres that provide nourishment for good gut flora. Prebiotic-rich foods include asparagus, bananas, leeks, onions, and garlic. Including them in your diet gives your probiotics the fuel they need to develop and function.

▪ **Moderate Sugar and Processed Food Consumption:** Overindulging in sugar and processed meals might upset the gut microbiome's delicate equilibrium. These meals could encourage the development of dangerous bacteria, which would cause inflammation and damage to the gut flora. For a healthy stomach, cut less on sugary snacks, drinks, and highly processed meals.

▪ **Include Fermented Foods:** Fermented foods are a natural source of probiotics that help maintain a balanced microbiota in the gut. Add miso, yoghourt, kefir, sauerkraut, and kimchi to your diet. These meals increase the variety of your gut microbiota by introducing living beneficial bacteria.

Mindful Eating Techniques: Developing mindful eating techniques may improve digestion. Chew everything slowly, enjoy every meal, and pay attention to your body's signals of hunger and fullness. Eating with awareness promotes healthy gut flora and optimum nutrition absorption.

▪ **Keep Yourself Hydrated:** Gut health depends on getting enough water. Water is essential for preserving the intestinal mucosal lining, which facilitates food transit through the digestive system. Drink enough water throughout the day to maintain the proper hydration and functionality of your stomach.

Why Probiotics Are Important

Overview of Probiotics

When ingested in sufficient quantities, probiotics—live microorganisms, mostly beneficial bacteria—offer health advantages. These microbes support a robust and healthy digestive system by adding to the variety and balance of the gut microbiome.

- **Enhancing Gut microbiota Diversity:** Research shows that improved health outcomes are linked to a more varied gut microbiota. Probiotics provide helpful strains of bacteria, which add to this variety. This variety improves the microbiome's capacity to carry out a number of tasks, including immunological support, nutrition absorption, and pathogen protection.

- **Controlling Immune Function:** Probiotics support the body's defensive mechanism, which is mostly dependent on the gut. Probiotics support the generation of antibodies, increase immune cell activity, and serve as a barrier against infections to assist regulate immunological function.

- **Supporting Digestive Health:** By preserving a healthy intestinal environment, probiotics help to support digestive health. They aid in the digestion of food, the synthesis of vital nutrients, and the control of dangerous bacterial overgrowth. Additionally, probiotics may lessen the symptoms of gastrointestinal conditions including inflammatory bowel disease (IBD) and irritable bowel syndrome (IBS).

- **Handling Antibiotic-Related Imbalances:** Although necessary for treating infections, antibiotics have the potential to upset the gut microbiome's equilibrium. Probiotic supplements aid in the restoration of beneficial bacteria populations both during and after antibiotic usage, avoiding antibiotic-associated diarrhoea and hastening the restoration of gut health.

- **Benefits for Mood and Mental Health:** New study points to a connection between probiotics and mental health. The gut-brain axis, which links the central nervous system with the gut, affects mood and mental processes. Probiotics may have a beneficial effect on this axis and help lessen symptoms of depression, anxiety, and stress.

Water for Digestive Health

Keeping the Integrity of the Gut Lining:
Sustaining the intestinal mucosal lining requires enough water. By acting as a barrier, this lining keeps dangerous chemicals out of the circulation. Maintaining the integrity of this

barrier with enough hydration promotes gut health in general.

- **Encouraging Nutrient Absorption:** Water is essential for the breakdown and assimilation of nutrients. It makes food particles easier to break down and flow through the digestive system. Hydrated intestines provide the best possible absorption of nutrients, which supply vital components for general well-being.

- **Preventing Constipation:** By making faeces more difficult to pass, dehydration may exacerbate constipation. Maintaining a healthy gut transit time, avoiding constipation, and encouraging regular bowel movements are all facilitated by drinking enough water.

- **Supporting Beneficial Bacteria:** Water is necessary for the gut's beneficial bacteria to survive and proliferate. It contributes to a balanced and healthy gut microbiota by fostering an environment that is favourable to the development of these microbes.

- **Improving Detoxification:** Drinking enough water helps the kidneys and liver do their part in the detoxification process. Hydration lessens the strain on these organs and creates a cleaner internal environment by washing away waste products and toxins, which indirectly improves gut health.

Chapter 3

intestine health and weight loss

While there are many different tactics to consider while starting a weight reduction journey, the relationship between gut health and weight control is one that is receiving more and more attention. Here, we'll examine the complex connection between gut health and weight reduction, comprehend the physiological processes involved, and discover easy weight loss techniques based on gut-centric approaches.

Knowing the Relationship

- **Gut Microbiome's Function:**

The large population of bacteria that live in the digestive system and are known as the gut microbiota is essential to metabolism and controlling body weight. Research has shown that people with varying body weights have distinct variances in the makeup of their gut microbiome. Both weight management and a more effective metabolism are linked to a diversified and well-balanced microbiota.

- **Impact on Reduction of Appetite:** The gut-brain axis allows the stomach and brain to connect, which affects satiety and hunger. An influence on hormones that regulate hunger is caused by signalling molecules produced by some gut bacteria. The disruption of this communication may result in overeating and weight gain due to an imbalance in the makeup of gut flora.

- **Influence on Nutrition Absorption:** A balanced gut microbiota improves nutrition absorption, which promotes general health. As a result of nutrient malabsorption brought on by an unbalanced microbiota, one may experience overindulgence and cravings as a means of making up for dietary inadequacies.

- **Prolonged inflammation:** Prolonged inflammation in the gastrointestinal tract has been associated with obesity and increased body weight. The body's calorie storage and use patterns may be changed by inflammation, which encourages the buildup of fat. The key to stopping inflammatory processes that lead to extra weight is to keep your gut environment balanced.

- **The Gut Microbiota Affects Insulin Sensitivity:** An important aspect of metabolic health is insulin sensitivity. Insulin resistance, which raises blood sugar levels and increases fat accumulation, may be a result of microbiota imbalances. Insulin sensitivity and metabolic efficiency may both be improved by restoring intestinal homeostasis.

No-Hass Weight Loss Strategies

Rank Foods High in Fiber First:
The key to losing weight and maintaining intestinal health is eating a diet high in fibre. Good-for-you foods that are high in fibre, such whole grains, fruits, vegetables, and legumes, help you feel fuller for less calories overall. A varied and healthy gut microbiota is also supported by fibre.

Opt for Foods High in Probiotics:

Non-digestible fibres called prebiotics nourish good microorganisms in the stomach. Prebiotic foods include foods like asparagus, bananas, leeks, onions, and garlic. You may encourage a healthy gut microbiota by including them into your diet, which will help probiotics develop and perform.

- **Include Probiotics:** They help maintain a healthy gut microbiota and may be found in fermented foods such as kimchi, kefir, yoghourt, and sauerkraut. Their function is to regulate metabolism and to increase the variety of gut flora. Weight control may be aided by consuming foods or supplements high in probiotics.

- **Practices for Mindful Eating:** Mindful eating may help with weight reduction by preventing overeating. Slowly chew your meal, pay attention to your body's signals of hunger and fullness, and enjoy every taste. Making more deliberate food choices is facilitated by mindful eating, which strengthens your relationship with your body's cues.

- **Drink Plenty of Water:** Losing weight requires adequate hydration. One way to decrease the risk of overeating is to feel fuller after drinking water before meals. Maintaining hydration also helps with waste product removal and promotes general metabolic processes.

- **Consistent Exercise:** Exercise on a regular basis is essential for weight reduction and intestinal health. The variety of the gut microbiome is increased by exercise, which has a beneficial impact on metabolism. For all-around health advantages, try to combine aerobic and strength training activities.

- **Cut Back on Processed Foods and Added Sugars:** These items might harm your digestive system and make you gain weight. Frequently deficient in vital nutrients, these meals could exacerbate inflammation. To help promote a healthy gut and aid in weight reduction, choose full, nutrient-dense meals.

A healthy weight and general well-being are directly correlated with getting quality sleep. Hormones that control appetite are upset when a person doesn't get enough sleep, which increases desires and makes overeating more likely. Make getting enough sleep a priority if you want to help yourself lose weight.

- **Control Stress:** Prolonged stress may undermine gut health and lead to weight gain. Mitigate the effects of stress on the mind and body by engaging in stress-reduction practices like yoga, deep breathing exercises, or meditation.

It is possible to simply attain and maintain a healthy weight by understanding the complex link between intestinal health and weight reduction. People may maximise their physical and digestive well-being while starting a comprehensive weight reduction journey by putting these suggestions into practice and maintaining a healthy gut microbiota.

Chapter 4

Using Gut Health to Release Stress

Stress is now a common companion for many people in our fast-paced and demanding world. Nonetheless, a viable approach to controlling and reducing the negative effects of stress on our wellbeing is provided by the complex relationship between gut health and stress levels. This section will examine how gut health affects stress and go into practical methods for reducing stress by maintaining a healthy gut.

How Stress Levels Are Affected by Gut Health

- **The Axis of Gut and Brain:**

The complex network of communication known as the gut-brain axis is central to the gut-stress relationship. The gut and the central nervous system can affect one another thanks to this two-way communication system. Through the vagus nerve, the gut connects to the brain and generates neurotransmitters that are essential for controlling mood and stress response.

- **The production of neurotransmitters and the microbiota**: The microbiota is a group of trillions of bacteria that live in the gut. Gamma-aminobutyric acid (GABA) and serotonin are two neurotransmitters that are actively produced by this diverse community of bacteria. Often referred to as the "feel-good" neurotransmitter, serotonin is important for mood regulation. The synthesis of these neurotransmitters can be interfered with by an imbalance in gut flora, which can affect stress levels and emotional health.

- **Cortisol**, also referred to as the stress hormone, is influenced by the hypothalamic-pituitary-adrenal (HPA) axis. A prolonged period of stress can dysregulate the HPA axis, which causes the overproduction of cortisol. This axis is influenced by the gut, and an unbalanced microbiome in the gut may lead to high cortisol levels, which worsen the stress response.

- **Stress and Inflammation**: A major factor in the relationship between stress and the gut is chronic inflammation, which is frequently linked to an unbalanced gut. The stress response can be triggered by signals sent from the gut to the brain by inflammation. There is a cyclical relationship between stress and gut health because stress-induced inflammation in the gut can further upset its balance.

Techniques for Reducing Stress

Practices of Mindful Eating:

Stress reduction and gut health can both be enhanced by practising mindful eating. Savour the tastes and textures of each bite while eating by concentrating on the sensory experience of it. When eating, stay away from screens and work-related activities. Eating with awareness improves digestion and creates a more balanced gut-brain axis.

Foods High in Probiotics: Including foods high in probiotics in your diet helps maintain a balanced gut microbiome, which affects the production of neurotransmitters and the stress response. Probiotic-rich foods include kefir, kimchi, sauerkraut, and yoghurt. Eating these foods offers a delicious and natural way to support stress resilience and nourish your gut.

Prebiotics for Gut Nourishment: Prebiotics are indigestible fibres that provide sustenance to good gut flora. These bacteria are encouraged to grow by foods high in prebiotics, like garlic, onions, and bananas. Maintaining a healthy gut microbiome through diet includes prebiotics, which may help balance out imbalances brought on by stress.

Frequent Exercise: Exercise is a powerful method for relieving stress and has a positive impact on gut health. Exercise decreases inflammation and encourages a diverse gut microbiome. Take part in something you enjoy doing; it could be yoga, dancing, or a brisk walk. A robust reaction to stress is promoted by the mutually reinforcing effects of exercise and gut health.

- **The parasympathetic nervous system:** This can be activated by combining deep breathing exercises and relaxation techniques, which can help induce a calm state of mind. Stress reduction techniques include diaphragmatic breathing, progressive muscle relaxation, and meditation. The gut-brain axis can perform at its best when stress levels decrease.

- **Adequate Sleep Hygiene:** Make maintaining proper sleep hygiene a top priority for stress reduction and gut health. A comfortable sleep environment should be created, a regular sleep schedule should be followed, and stimulants like caffeine should be avoided right before bed. Restorative sleep improves the body's capacity to handle stress and aids in the repair of the intestinal lining.

- **Herbal Teas with Relaxing Effects**: Some herbal teas, like peppermint and chamomile, have relaxing qualities that can lower stress levels and improve gut health. These teas have the potential to ease digestive issues and encourage rest. Warm herbal tea can be a simple yet powerful ritual for relieving stress.

- **Limiting Alcohol and Caffeine Intake:** Excessive alcohol and caffeine consumption can aggravate gut health and increase stress. Cortisol levels can rise and sleep patterns can be disrupted by both drugs. The secret to keeping things in balance is to moderate intake and pay attention to how they affect the gut and stress response.

- **Mind-Body Exercises:** Taking part in mind-body exercises, like yoga or tai chi, promotes a comprehensive strategy for stress reduction. By combining movement, breath awareness, and mindfulness, these techniques help people relax and lessen the physiological effects of stress on the digestive system.

It is possible to develop comprehensive well-being strategies by comprehending the profound relationship between gut health and stress liberation. People can cultivate resilience in their gut and their reaction to stress by embracing mindful eating practices, incorporating foods that nourish the gut, learning stress-relieving techniques, and advocating for a harmonious lifestyle.

Chapter 5

Digestive Harmony: A Comprehensive Guide to Promoting Wellness

Achieving digestive balance is critical to general health. In addition to facilitating the effective breakdown and absorption of nutrients, a healthy digestive system also supports the body's resiliency and vitality. In this section, we will examine various foods that support the maintenance of digestive harmony as well as strategies for promoting digestive wellness.

Aiming to Encourage Digestive Health

- **The Basis of Hydration:**

The health of the digestive system depends on adequate hydration. Water makes it easier for food to pass through the digestive system smoothly, which helps to encourage regular bowel movements and avoid constipation. Maintaining a healthy gut environment also involves drinking enough water to support the integrity of the mucosal lining of the intestines.

- **A diet high in fibre promotes regularity:**

Gut health is largely dependent on dietary fibre. It prevents constipation and encourages regular bowel movements by giving the stool more bulk. Good sources of fibre include whole grains, fruits, vegetables, nuts, and seeds. A diverse range of fibre types are ensured when you incorporate these foods into your diet, which promotes digestive harmony.

- **Probiotics and Gut Balance:** Probiotics are good bacteria that help maintain a balanced gut microbiome. Probiotic-rich foods like kefir, yoghourt, sauerkraut, and kimchi introduce live cultures that support a healthy gut environment and help break down food. Probiotics support immune function and provide defence against pathogenic microorganisms.

- **Benefiting Gut Bacteria with Prebiotics:** Prebiotics are indigestible fibres that provide sustenance for the good bacteria in the stomach. These bacteria are encouraged to grow by foods high in prebiotics, such as onions, garlic, bananas, and asparagus. Keeping the microbiome healthy and supporting overall digestive well-being requires a consistent supply of prebiotics.

- **Digestive Enzymes:** In order for the body to absorb nutrients from food, digestive enzymes are necessary for efficient digestion. Natural enzymes found in some foods aid in digestion even though the body produces its own enzymes. Bromelain and papain, for instance, are found in pineapple and papaya, respectively, and they help in the digestion of proteins.

- **Herbs for Calm Digestion:** You can help your digestive system feel more at ease by including calming herbs in your routine. For example, the anti-inflammatory qualities of peppermint and ginger can help reduce indigestion symptoms. Easy ways to incorporate these herbs into your diet are to drink ginger tea or add fresh mint to meals.

- **Chew Food Mindfully:** Since the mouth is where digestion starts, chewing mindfully is essential to supporting digestive health. Food is more easily broken down into smaller particles by chewing it thoroughly, which facilitates further digestion and nutrient absorption by stomach enzymes. Furthermore, chewing with awareness transmits signals to the brain that support optimal digestive function.

- **Control Stress for Gut Health:** Prolonged stress can disrupt the gut-brain axis, which can have a detrimental effect on digestion. Stress can worsen the symptoms of indigestion and contribute to the development of disorders like irritable bowel syndrome (IBS). A calm and balanced digestive system can be achieved by incorporating stress-reduction methods like yoga, deep breathing, and meditation.

Foods to Promote Digestion

- **Yogurt.**

Live cultures of beneficial bacteria are found in yoghurt, making it a food high in probiotics. These microorganisms assist digestion and maintain a balanced gut microbiome. To get the most out of your yoghurt, go for plain, unsweetened varieties. You can also add fresh fruit or a drizzle of honey for flavour.

- **Ginger:** Related to its calming effects on the digestive tract, ginger possesses anti-inflammatory qualities. Ginger can help relieve indigestion and nausea symptoms whether it is drunk as a tea, added to food, or eaten raw.

- **Peppermint:** Peppermint has a relaxing effect on the gastrointestinal system and can help reduce indigestion and IBS symptoms. For a cooling and easy-on-the-digestive addition, sip peppermint tea or add fresh mint leaves to salads and other dishes.

- **Papaya:** The enzyme papain, which is found in papayas, helps break down proteins. Papaya can help promote effective protein digestion and nutrient absorption in your diet. Savour fresh papaya as a snack or incorporate it into fruit salads for a touch of the tropics.

- **Pineapple:** Bromelain, an enzyme found in pineapples, aids in the digestion of proteins. Whether you eat pineapple raw or in fruit salads and smoothies, it can help with digestion and improve the health of your gut in general.

- **Bananas:** Packed with dietary fibre and prebiotics to support good gut flora, bananas are a power food. Additionally, they are easily digested, which makes them a gentle option for people with sensitive stomachs. Bananas can be eaten as a snack or added to breakfast bowls and smoothies.

- **Whole Grains:** Packed full of fibre, whole grains like quinoa, brown rice, and oats help to maintain regular bowel motions and digestive health. In addition to contributing to a balanced diet, these grains offer long-lasting energy. To get the most nutritional benefits, choose whole grains over refined grains.

- **Fennel:** Fennel has long been used as a digestive aid, particularly for indigestion and bloating. Fennel seeds' aromatic compounds have the potential to ease digestive tract tension. For enhanced flavour and support for your digestive system, try making fennel tea or adding the seeds to your food.

▪ **Bone broth:** Packed with nutrients and collagen, bone broth is good for the health of your digestive system. A healthy gut environment is promoted by the minerals and amino acids in bone broth, which also support the lining of the digestive tract. You can enjoy bone broth on its own or use it as a base for soups and stews.

▪ **Pulses and Legumes:** Rich in fibre and protein, pulses and legumes comprise beans, lentils, and chickpeas. They support regular bowel movements and supply vital nutrients, which both support digestive wellness. When planning meals, incorporate a range of pulses to promote a nutrient-dense, gut-friendly diet.

A holistic approach, digestive harmony entails mindful eating, adding foods that are good for the gut, and embracing lifestyle choices that promote general wellbeing. People may support a robust and well-balanced digestive system by drinking enough water, eating a diet high in fibre, taking probiotics and prebiotics, and selecting foods that facilitate easy digestion.

Chapter 6

Using Gut Health to Reduce Inflammation

Chronic inflammation may be troublesome even though it's a normal and necessary component of the body's defensive system. A potential approach to controlling and reducing inflammation is provided by the complex link between gut health and inflammation. This section will examine the relationship between gut health and inflammation, elucidating the underlying processes and delving into anti-inflammatory foods and activities that promote general health.

Inflammation and Gut Health

- **Inflammation and the Gut Microbiota:**
Inflammation is mostly regulated by the gut microbiome, a complex community of billions of bacteria that live in the digestive system. In a state of equilibrium, the immune system reacts to threats correctly without inducing excessive inflammation. This is made possible by a balanced and diversified microbiome.

- **Inflammation and Leaky Gut Syndrome:**
Chronic inflammation may be exacerbated by leaky gut syndrome, a condition in which the integrity of the gut lining is damaged. Toxins, germs, and partially digested food particles may all enter the circulation when the lining becomes porous. This sets off an immunological reaction that causes inflammation all across the body.

- **Microbial Diversity and Inflammatory Diseases:** Research indicates that a number of inflammatory illnesses are linked to a decrease in gut microbial diversity. A lack of variety may make it more difficult for the microbiome to carry out vital tasks like immune response regulation and gut barrier integrity maintenance. Inflammatory problems may arise and worsen as a result of this imbalance.

- **Inflammation and the Gut-Brain Axis:**
Inflammation is influenced by the gut-brain axis, a two-way communication pathway between the stomach and the central neurological system. Inflammatory reactions in the gut may be influenced by stress, which is a role in dysregulation of the gut-brain axis. On the other hand, gut inflammation has the ability to communicate with the brain and may have an impact on mood and cognitive abilities.

Meals and Activities that Reduce Inflammation

- **Fatty Acids Omega-3:**

Rich sources of omega-3 fatty acids, such as sardines, mackerel, and salmon, have strong anti-inflammatory qualities. These fatty acids aid in the synthesis of chemicals that reduce inflammation and serve to modulate the body's inflammatory response. Consuming a diet high in omega-3-rich foods promotes both general health and gastrointestinal health.

- **Turmeric and Curcumin:** Curcumin is a molecule with potent anti-inflammatory properties that is found in turmeric, a spice that is often used in traditional medicine. It has been shown that curcumin modulates inflammatory pathways, which may help reduce the symptoms associated with inflammatory disorders. Reducing inflammation may be achieved by adding turmeric to food or by supplementing with curcumin.

- **Brightly Colored Fruits and Vegetables:** The vivid hues of fruits and vegetables indicate the presence of phytochemicals and antioxidants that reduce inflammation. Antioxidants found in leafy greens, tomatoes, berries, and cherries help squelch inflammation and counteract free radical damage. Including a selection of vibrant vegetables in your diet encourages the production of several anti-inflammatory chemicals.

- **Foods Rich in Probiotics:** Fermented foods such as kefir, kimchi, and yoghurt contain probiotics, which are helpful bacteria that support gut health and may also have anti-inflammatory properties. These microbes assist in maintaining a healthy gut environment and regulate the immune system. Eating meals high in probiotics helps maintain healthy digestion and reduce inflammation.

▪ **Green Tea**: Green tea has anti-inflammatory qualities due to its polyphenols, especially epigallocatechin gallate (EGCG). Drinking green tea on a regular basis might improve general health and aid lower inflammation. Selecting green tea as a beverage offers possible anti-inflammatory advantages in addition to hydration.

▪ **Ginger**: Because of its anti-inflammatory qualities, ginger has been utilised for ages. It has ingredients including gingerol, which may help reduce inflammation and ease the signs and symptoms of inflammatory diseases. For reducing inflammation, adding fresh ginger to food, drinking ginger tea, or taking pills may all be helpful.

- **olive oil:** Extra virgin olive oil is high in monounsaturated fats and includes substances that reduce inflammation. Olive oil intake has been linked to a decrease in the body's inflammatory marker levels. To maximise olive oil's anti-inflammatory properties, use it as your main cooking oil and in salad dressings.

Nuts and Seeds: Packed full of antioxidants and omega-3 fatty acids, nuts and seeds like flaxseed, walnuts, and almonds are great sources of nutrients that reduce inflammation. A nutrient-dense and enjoyable strategy to reduce inflammation in your diet is to include a variety of nuts and seeds.

- **Appropriate Hydration:** Retaining intestinal health and controlling inflammation need proper hydration. Water helps maintain the intestinal mucosal lining, which creates a barrier that keeps dangerous things out. To enhance general well-being and encourage hydration, make it a goal to consume enough water throughout the day.

- **Meditation and Stress Reduction:** Stress reduction techniques are crucial for general health as they reduce inflammation, which is a result of chronic stress. Inflammation may be decreased by modulating the body's stress response with the use of deep breathing techniques, yoga, mindfulness, and meditation. Making relaxation techniques a priority promotes digestive health as well as mental wellbeing.

Choosing foods, leading a healthy lifestyle, and emphasising general wellbeing are all part of a multidimensional strategy to reduce inflammation via gut health. People may maintain a robust and balanced immune system by making educated decisions by being aware of the complex relationship between inflammation and the gut flora.

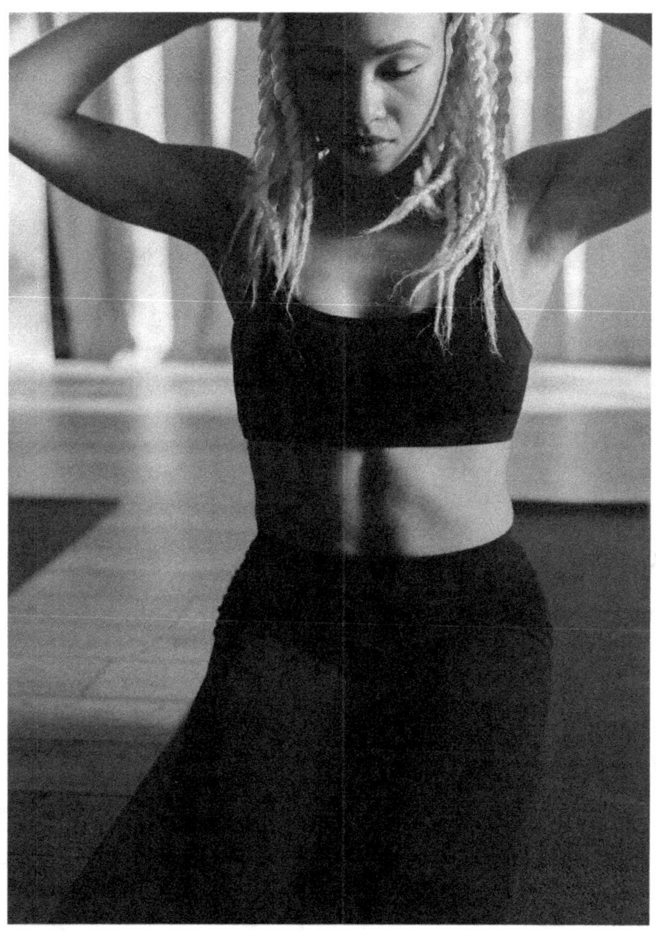

Chapter 7

Discovering the Secrets to Being Your Best Self

Setting out on a quest to become your greatest self is a comprehensive undertaking that takes into account your mental, bodily, and spiritual well-being. We will look at a holistic approach to health in this part, highlighting the connections between many facets of our life. We'll also explore the transforming power of mindfulness, which is essential to learning the keys to being your best self.

Holistic Perspective on Health

▪ **Mind-Body Reconnection:**

Understanding the complex relationship between the mind and body is central to the idea of holistic health. Our mental health, feelings, and thoughts have a significant impact on our physical health. On the other hand, our mental and emotional moods may be influenced by our physical health. Accepting a holistic viewpoint entails fostering both facets in order to attain total wellbeing.

- **Food as Fuel for Body and Mind:** Mindful eating is the first step in a comprehensive approach to health. Food supplies vital nutrients that assist mental and emotional health in addition to serving as the body's fuel. In addition to ensuring that your body gets the nutrition it needs for optimum functioning, eating a balanced, diverse diet high in whole foods also helps to promote mental clarity and emotional stability.

- **Physical Exercise for Vitality:** A fundamental component of holistic health is frequent physical exercise. In addition to building muscle, exercise releases endorphins, the "feel-good" chemicals that improve mood. Finding enjoyment in physical activity, whether it be via yoga, strength training, or brisk walking, is beneficial to one's physical and emotional health.

- **Restorative Sleep:** The value of restorative sleep for the body and mind is recognized by holistic health. The body goes through important activities like hormone control, memory consolidation, and tissue repair when you sleep. Making enough sleep a priority is essential to reaching optimum health in all respects.

- **Social Cohesion and Emotional Welfare:** Since humans are social animals, our interactions have a big impact on our general well-being. Emotional resilience and mental health are enhanced by creating and sustaining strong social ties. Building caring connections that provide emotional support and a feeling of community is crucial to holistic wellness.

- **Stress Reduction and Mental Sturdiness:** Prolonged stress may have a significant negative impact on one's bodily and mental well-being. In order to support mental resilience, a comprehensive approach incorporates efficient stress-reduction techniques. People may manage stress and keep a balanced viewpoint by using strategies like deep breathing exercises, mindfulness, and meditation.

- **Environmental Wellness:** A holistic approach to health considers not only one's own well-being but also that of the environment. A key component of a holistic approach is understanding the connection between the health of the planet and human health. Choosing environmentally friendly options, minimising negative effects on the environment, and spending time in nature all enhance general wellbeing.

- **Spiritual Satisfaction:** A vital component of holistic health is spiritual well-being, which is very individualised. It entails cultivating an inner feeling of calm, connecting with one's ideals, and finding meaning and purpose in life. This aspect of health is unique to each person and might include transcendental activities, meditation, prayer, or other practices.

Mindfulness Included

The definition of mindfulness is "a state of active, open attention to the present moment." It entails embracing ideas and emotions as they are, without passing judgement on them. By incorporating mindfulness into your everyday routine, you may develop a more acute awareness of the present moment and a stronger connection with the people and things around you.

▪ **Mindful Eating Practices:** Mindful eating is one method to incorporate awareness. Take your time and enjoy every mouthful of your food, focusing on its tastes, textures, and feelings rather than speeding through it. In addition to improving the eating experience, mindful eating encourages better meal selections and facilitates digestion.

- **Movement with attention:** When physical activity is undertaken with attention, it takes on more significance. Mindful movement, whether it is yoga, walking, or any other kind of exercise, is being totally present in the doing. Observe your breath, your body's feelings, and your surroundings. This improves the workout's efficacy and offers a psychological reprieve from the stresses of everyday life.

- **Mindfulness Meditation:** great technique for developing awareness and fostering mental clarity is mindfulness meditation. Locate a peaceful area, take a comfortable seat, and concentrate on your breathing or a particular object of interest. As ideas come to mind, just bring your attention back to the here and now while acknowledging them without passing judgement. Frequent mindfulness meditation may improve attention, lower stress levels, and improve emotional health.

- **Exercises for Mindful Breathing:** Mindful breathing is a basic yet powerful mindfulness method. Throughout the day, set aside some time to breathe deeply and intentionally. Pay attention to how your body feels as the breath comes in and goes out. By assisting in the nervous system's regulation, mindful breathing fosters serenity and lessens the negative effects of stress.

Incorporate mindfulness into your everyday routine by giving each job your whole attention. Engage in the present moment whenever you can, whether it be while working, walking, or doing the dishes. In addition to improving the quality of your deeds, this practice fosters awareness of the present moment and an appreciation for life's little pleasures.

- **Using Mindfulness to Control Emotions:** Mindfulness is an effective strategy for controlling emotions. When confronted with difficult emotions, stop for a while and observe without responding right away. Accept the feelings and give them permission to exist in their current state without passing judgement. This attentive approach may promote a more balanced response to emotional situations and help avoid impulsive responses.

- **Utilising Technology Mindfully:** In the digital era, keeping a healthy balance while using technology requires integrating mindfulness. Make a conscious decision about how much time you spend on screens. Take pauses to engage in mindful breathing or just to be in the moment. Setting limits while using technology promotes mental health and a more deliberate way of living.

Developing a holistic approach to health and incorporating mindfulness into all areas of your life are essential steps towards unlocking the secrets of becoming your greatest self. People may be on a transforming journey toward optimum well-being by realising the interdependence of mind, body, and spirit.

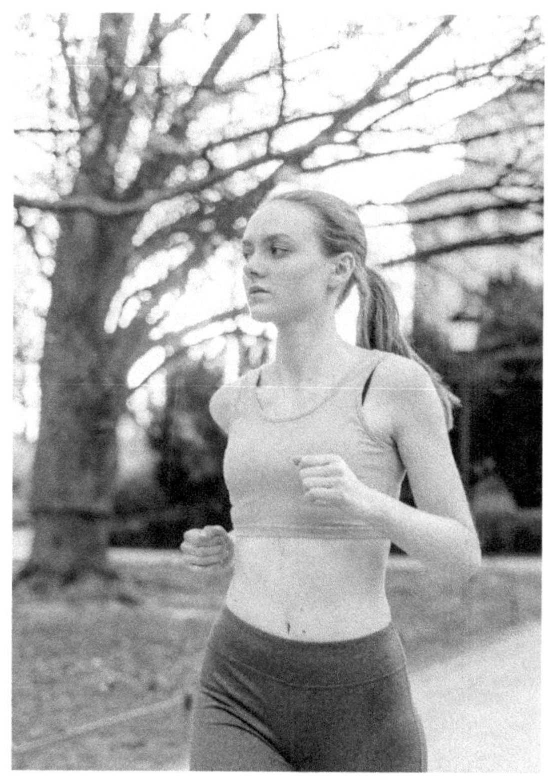

Chapter 8

The Relationship Between Gut and Emotion

The relationship between intestinal health and emotional well-being is critical to the quest of a happy and fulfilled life. This section delves into the complex link between the stomach and emotions, examining the ways in which our gut health might affect our overall happiness and mood. We'll also explore happy living techniques and provide doable solutions for recovering joy in every second of life.

Gut Health's Significance for Emotional Wellness

- **The Axis of the Gut and Brain:**

An important factor in the relationship between gut health and emotional well-being is the gut-brain axis, a bidirectional communication network that links the stomach and the brain. The stomach may affect emotional reactions and vice versa because of this connection that takes place via neurological, hormonal, and immune pathways.

- **stomach Production of Serotonin:** Often referred to as the "feel-good" neurotransmitter, serotonin is mostly produced in the stomach. Serotonin is released by the lining of the gastrointestinal system and subsequently affects mood control. An unbalanced population of gut bacteria may affect the synthesis of serotonin, which may be linked to mood disorders including sadness and anxiety.

- **Emotional Resilience and Gut Microbiota Diversity:** The billions of bacteria that make up the gut microbiota are a major factor in emotional resilience. Better mental health outcomes are linked to a microbiome that is rich and varied. On the other hand, emotional problems may be exacerbated by a disturbed microbiota, which is often brought on by things like antibiotic usage or an unbalanced diet.

- **Chronic inflammation** in the stomach has been related to mood problems and a diminished feeling of overall well being. Neurotransmitters and brain circuits involved in mood regulation may be affected by inflammatory indicators. To promote emotional balance, it becomes imperative to address gut inflammation via dietary and lifestyle choices.

- **Stress and gut health:** There is a reciprocal association between stress and gut health.

Dysbiosis may result from long-term stress upsetting the gut microbiota's equilibrium. However, an unbalanced stomach may communicate with the brain in a way that intensifies the stress reaction. Stress management techniques are advantageous for both emotional and gastrointestinal health.

Activities that Promote Joyful Living

- **Intentional Consumption to Promote Gut-Emotion Equilibrium:**
Accept mindful eating as a way to improve your mental and digestive health. Savour each piece of food mindfully and without interruption, focusing on the sensory experience. Eating mindfully encourages good digestion, which

improves gut-brain axis function and elevates happiness.

▪ **Probiotics for Emotional Resilience:** Include foods high in probiotics in your diet to help maintain a healthy gut microbiota. Probiotic-rich foods include kombucha, sauerkraut, kefir, and yoghurt. These healthy bacteria support emotional resilience and are involved in the synthesis of serotonin. A tasty and proactive step toward joyful life might be adding probiotics to your diet.

▪ **Prebiotics:** Nondigestible fibres that support good gut flora are known as prebiotics, and they are crucial for preserving gut health. Prebiotics are abundant in foods including asparagus, bananas, onions, and garlic. By promoting the development of advantageous bacteria in your diet, you may create a healthy gut environment and perhaps improve your mental well-being.

- **Frequent Physical Exercise for Mood Enhancement:** Being physically active on a daily basis is a great way to support gut health and happy feelings. Exercise helps maintain a healthy gut flora and produces endorphins, the body's natural mood enhancers. Make exercise a fun part of your routine by finding activities you like, such as dancing, walking, or cycling.

- **Good Sleep:** Prioritise getting a good night's sleep as the cornerstone of emotional recovery. The body performs vital functions that affect mood control while we sleep. Aim for enough sleep each night, establish a regular sleep schedule, and provide a cosy sleeping space. Restful sleep promotes emotional well-being and digestive health.

- **For Gut-Emotion Harmony, Get in Touch with Nature:**

Reduced stress and an enhanced mood have been related to spending time in nature. Exposure to nature enhances variety and equilibrium in the gut microbiome. Whether it's via gardening, a stroll in the park, or just spending time outside, take some time to connect with nature.

- **Using Mindfulness Meditation to Promote Emotional Equilibrium:** Incorporate mindfulness meditation into your everyday schedule to foster emotional equilibrium. Research has shown that engaging in mindfulness activities, such as focused breathing and present-moment awareness, may lower stress and improve gut health. Make time for mindfulness meditation every day and let it develop into a life-changing routine.

- **Develop Good Social ties:** Emotional health is greatly enhanced by having positive social ties. Build happy and fulfilling connections in your life. Emphasise genuine relationships that provide support and promote a feeling of belonging, whether via in-person or internet contacts.

- **Show Gratitude for Emotional Upliftment:** Gratitude is a powerful tool for improving emotional health. Spend a moment every day expressing your thankfulness for all that is good in your life. This easy exercise helps to cultivate an attitude of wealth and pleasure by turning attention from the negative to the good. To record instances of thankfulness, think about starting a gratitude notebook.

- **Take Part in Happy Hobbies and Activities:** Find and do things that make you happy and give you a feeling of accomplishment. Make time for things that align with your interests, whether they be artistic endeavours, hobbies, or quality time with loved ones. Happy memories support good feelings and a healthy gut-brain axis.

Realising the close relationship between intestinal health and mental well-being is essential to recovering delight in every moment. People may improve their emotional resilience and general well-being by putting into practice habits that promote a healthy gut microbiota, such as mindful eating, including probiotics and prebiotics, and engaging in regular physical exercise.

Chapter 9

Healthy recipes for Super gut health for women

Breakfast Blitz

1. Probiotics Parfait:

Overview: For a delicious and gut-friendly breakfast, pair probiotic-rich yoghurt with crisp granola and fresh berries.

Five minutes in total
One serving

Ingredients :

• One cup of probiotic-rich Greek yoghourt

• Half a cup of high-fibre granola

•1/2 cup mixed berries, including strawberries and blueberries

• One spoonful of maple syrup or honey

Directions:

1.Arrange Greek yoghurt, granola, and mix 2. berries in a glass or dish.

2.Drizzle with maple syrup or honey.

3. Repeat layers and enjoy.

Nutritional information

350 calories

20g of protein

8g of fibre

Probiotics: Vary according on yoghourt variety

2. Chia Seed Pudding

Overview: A quick and healthy pudding to start the day that is full of fibre and omega-3 fatty acids.

Six hours total, including cooling time
Two servings:

Ingredients:
- One-fourth cup chia seeds
- One cup almond milk
- One tsp vanilla essence
- One spoonful of honey
- Fresh fruit to garnish

Directions:
1.Combine the almond milk, honey, vanilla essence, and chia seeds in a bowl.
2.Stir periodically and refrigerate for at least 6 hours or overnight.

3.Before serving, place a fresh fruit on top.

Nutritional information:

180 calories

5g of protein

10g of fibre

2.5g of omega-3 fatty acids

3. Omelette with avocado and spinach

Overview: A nutrient-dense omelette that has spinach, creamy avocado, and vitamins in moderation.

Ten minutes in total

One serving

Ingredients:

▪ two eggs

- sliced half an avocado and a handful of fresh spinach
- To taste, add salt and pepper.

One tsp olive oil

Directions:

1.Add salt and pepper to the eggs as you whisk them.

2.In a skillet with heated olive oil, add the spinach and cook until it wilts.

2.Over the spinach, pour the whisked eggs and simmer until set.

4.Scoop out the avocado slices, fold over, and

Nutritional information:

300 calories

15g of protein

20g of good fats

6g of fibre

4. Smoothie Bowl with Fruit and Yogurt

Overview: A nutritious start to your day with a delicious smoothie bowl filled with a blend of fruits and yoghourt high in probiotics.

Six minutes in total
One serving

Ingredients:

- 1/2 cup of probiotic-rich Greek yoghourt
- 1/2 cup of mixed berries, including raspberries and blueberries
- Half a banana, cut
- One-fourth cup granola
- One spoonful of butter made with almonds

Directions:

1.Blend half of the mixed berries with Greek yoghurt.

2.Transfer into a bowl, then garnish with almond butter, granola, banana slices, and the remaining berries.

Nutritional information:

380 calories

18g of protein

7g of fibre

Probiotics: Vary according to the kind of yoghurt.

5. Whole Grain Bread with Avocado Smashed

Overview: A simple yet filling breakfast of whole grain bread with mashed avocado, which is high in nutrients.

Five minutes in total

One serving

Ingredients:

- Two pieces of healthy grain bread, half an avocado, crushed cherry tomatoes, and optional red pepper flakes cut
- To taste, add salt and pepper.

Directions:

1.Toast pieces of whole grain bread until golden.

2.Over each piece, spread mashed avocado.

3.Add sliced cherry tomatoes, salt, pepper, and optional red pepper flakes on top.

Nutritional information:

280 calories

8g of protein

15g of good fats

Fibre: nine grams

6. Overnight Oats with Blueberries and Almonds

Overview: A tasty and satisfying breakfast that can be prepared ahead of time, with almonds, blueberries, and oats.

Six hours total, including cooling time
One serving

Ingredients:
- Half a cup of rolled oats
- half a cup of almond milk
- one-fourth cup blueberries
- One spoonful of butter made with almonds
- One tsp of chia seeds

Directions:

1.In a container, combine rolled oats, almond milk, chia seeds, blueberries, and almond butter.

2.Keep chilled for a minimum of six hours or overnight.

3.Before serving, give a quick stir and top with more almonds and blueberries.

Nutritional information:

320 calories

9g of protein

14g of good fats

10g of fibre

7. Breakfast Wrap with Spinach and Feta

Overview: A tasty way to start the day, this savoury breakfast wrap with eggs, feta cheese, and spinach is full of protein.

15 minutes in total

One serving

Ingredients:

- One tortilla made with whole grains
- two scrambled eggs
- A handful of fresh spinach
- Two teaspoons of crumbled feta cheese
- Hot sauce or salsa are optional.

Directions:

1.In a pan, cook scrambled eggs until fluffy.

2.Top with a layer of warm fresh spinach tortilla.

3.Top with crumbled feta cheese and scrambled eggs.

4.If desired, top with spicy sauce or salsa after rolling into a wrap.

Nutritional information:

350 calories

20g of protein

15g of good fats

5g of fibre

These healthy and delectable breakfast dishes provide a range of choices to promote gut health along with mouthwatering tastes to brighten your mornings. Adapt ingredients and portion quantities to suit each person's dietary requirements and preferences. Savour these nutrient-dense breakfast options as part of a healthy, well-balanced diet.

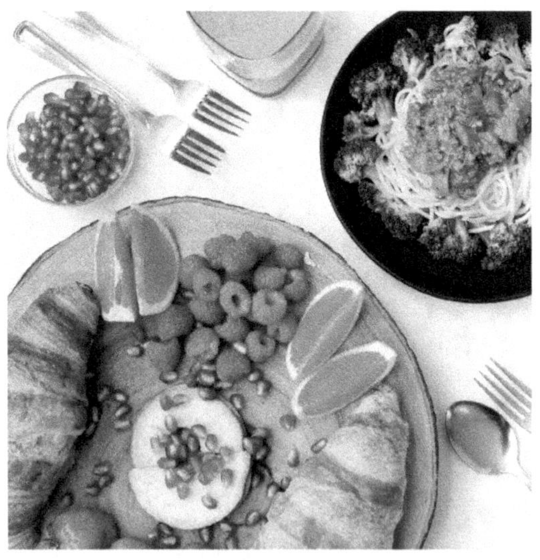

Lunch

1. Tofu with Veggies Buddha Bowl:

Overview: A filling and vibrant bowl of quinoa, mixed veggies, and a tasty dressing for a satisfying midday meal that is good for the stomach.

Thirty minutes total

2 servings

Ingredients:

- one cup of quinoa, cooked
- broccoli florets in one cup
- Halved cherry tomatoes (1/2 cup)
- half a cup of sliced cucumber
- Julienned half a cup of carrots
- 1/4 cup of hummus
- Two teaspoons of olive oil

- one tablespoon of lemon juice
- Add salt and pepper to taste.
- Garnish with fresh herbs if desired.

Directions:

1.Fill bowls with cooked quinoa.

2.After the broccoli is soft, steam or roast it and divide it among bowls.

3.Put carrots, cucumber, and cherry tomatoes in each bowl.

4.Combine hummus, olive oil, lemon juice, salt, and pepper in a small bowl. Pour over the bowls.

5.If desired, add fresh herbs as a garnish.

Nutritional information:

Four hundred calories

12 grams of protein

18g of healthy fats

8 grams of fibre

2. Salad with Avocado and Salmon

Overview: A tasty and gut-friendly lunch choice, this protein-rich salad has grilled salmon, avocado, and a zesty vinaigrette.

20 minutes in total

2 servings

Ingredients:

- Two pan-fried salmon fillets
- four cups of mixed greens
- Slicing one avocado and halving half of the cherry tomatoes
- Slicing 1/4 cup of red onion thinly
- Two teaspoons of olive oil

One-tsp balsamic vinegar

- One tsp dijon mustard
- Add salt and pepper to taste.
- Slices of lemon to serve

Directions:

1.Fill dishes with mixed greens.

2. Add red onion, cherry tomatoes, avocado slices, and cooked salmon on top.

3. Mix the olive oil, Dijon mustard, balsamic vinegar, salt, and pepper in a small bowl. Pour over the salad.

4. Serve with slices of lemon on the side.

Nutritional information:

Four hundred fifty calories

25 grams of protein

30 grams of good fats

Ten grams of fibre

3. Pasta Salad with Chickpeas

Overview: Thisvivid,Mediterranean-flavoured, high-protein chickpea salad is ideal for promoting intestinal health during lunch.

15 minutes in total.

4 Servings

Ingredients:

- Two drained and rinsed cans of chickpeas
- 1 cup cherry tomatoes, 1 cucumber cut in half, diced, 1/2 cup sliced Kalamata olives, 1/4 cup finely chopped red onion, and 1/4 cup crumbled feta cheese
- Three tsp olive oil
- Two teaspoons of vinegar made from red wine.
- One tsp. of dried oregano
- Add salt and pepper to taste.
- For garnish, use fresh parsley.

Directions:

1.Chickpeas, cucumber, red onion, olives, cherry tomatoes, and feta cheese should all be combined in a big dish.

2. Olive oil, red wine vinegar, dried oregano, salt, and pepper should all be combined in a small bowl.

3. Drizzle the salad with the dressing and toss to mix.

4. Before serving, sprinkle some fresh parsley on top.

Nutritional information:

350 Calories

15 grams of protein

18g of healthy fats

Ten grams of fibre

4. Vegetarian Sushi Bowl

Overview: A nutrient-dense and gut-friendly lunch alternative is this disassembled sushi bowl made with brown rice, veggies, and avocado.

Twenty-five minutes total

2 servings

Ingredients:

- one cup cooked brown rice

- one sliced avocado

- Julienned half a cup of cucumber

- Julienned half a cup of carrot

- 1/4 cup of ginger pickles

- Two tsp low-sodium soy sauce

- A single spoonful of rice vinegar

- A tsp of sesame oil

- To garnish, add sesame seeds.

- Seaweed (nori) strips for serving

Directions:

1.Evenly distribute cooked brown rice among bowls.

2. Place pieces of avocado, cucumber, and carrot over the rice.

3. Combine the rice vinegar, sesame oil, and soy sauce in a small bowl. Pour over the bowls.

4. Add pickled ginger, sesame seeds, and nori strips as garnish.

Nutritional information:

380 Calories

8 grams of protein

15 grams of good fats

Ten grams of fibre

5. Vegetable and Lentil Soup

Overview: This filling and satiating lunch dish is a robust, high-fibre lentil soup paired with a colourful vegetable medley.

Forty minutes in total

6 servings

Ingredients:

- 1 cup dry lentils, 1 onion, chopped, diced, sliced, and 3 cloves minced garlic, along with 2 carrots and 2 celery stalks
- one can of chopped tomatoes
- Six cups of low-sodium veggie broth
- One tsp cumin
- one tsp of turmeric
- Add salt and pepper to taste.
- For garnish, use fresh parsley.

Directions:

1.Saute the celery, carrots, onions, and garlic in a big saucepan until they are tender.

2.Add the lentils, diced tomatoes, turmeric, cumin, salt, and pepper, along with the

3.vegetable broth. Heat up till boiling.

4. Once the lentils are soft, reduce the heat and simmer for 30 minutes.

5. Before serving, sprinkle some fresh parsley on top.

Nutritional Information:

Two hundred fifty calories

15 grams of protein

Fibre: twelve grams

Iron: 0.4 mg

6. Quinoa salad with grilled chicken

Overview: A filling and healthy lunch may be made with this protein-rich salad that includes quinoa, grilled chicken, and an assortment of veggies.

Thirty minutes total

4 Servings

Ingredients:

- Two cups of prepared quinoa
- Grilled and cut one-pound chicken breast

- Two cups of mixed greens
- One cup of halved cherry tomatoes
- Half a cup of chopped cucumber
- Slicing 1/4 cup of red onion thinly
- 1/4 cup grated feta cheese
- Two teaspoons of olive oil
- One-tsp balsamic vinegar
- Add salt and pepper to taste.

Directions:

1.Toss together cooked quinoa, grilled chicken, cucumber, red onion, cherry tomatoes, and feta cheese in a big bowl.

2. Mix the balsamic vinegar, olive oil, salt, and pepper in a small bowl. Pour over the salad.

3. Serve after tossing to mix.

Nutritional information:

Four hundred and twenty-one calories

30 grams of protein

18g of healthy fats

8 grams of fibre

7. Vegetable Wrap with Roasted Roasts

Overview: A filling and gut-nourishing lunch, this wrap is full of flavour and made with whole-grain tortilla, hummus, and roasted veggies.

Twenty-five minutes total
2 servings

Ingredients:

- One slice of zucchini
- 1 sliced bell pepper
- 1 sliced red onion
- Two teaspoons of olive oil
- One tsp cumin

- One teaspoon of paprika

- Add salt and pepper to taste.

- 4 tacos made with whole grains

- half a cup of hummus

- Garnish with fresh herbs if desired.

Directions:

1.Preheat the oven to 200°C, or 400°F.

Add olive oil, cumin, paprika, salt, and 2. 2. 2. pepper to the bell pepper, red onion, and zucchini.

3. When the veggies are soft, roast them for 20 minutes in the oven.

4. Each whole-grain tortilla should be spread with hummus, then topped with roasted veggies and, if preferred, fresh herbs.

5. Serve after rolling into a wrap.

Nutritional information:

380 Calories

Protein: ten grams

18g of healthy fats

Ten grams of fibre

In addition to emphasising gut health, these lunch dishes include a range of tastes and minerals to sustain your energy levels throughout the day. Depending on dietary requirements and personal tastes, modify the ingredients and serving sizes. Savour these filling and tasty lunch options as part of a healthy, gut-friendly diet.

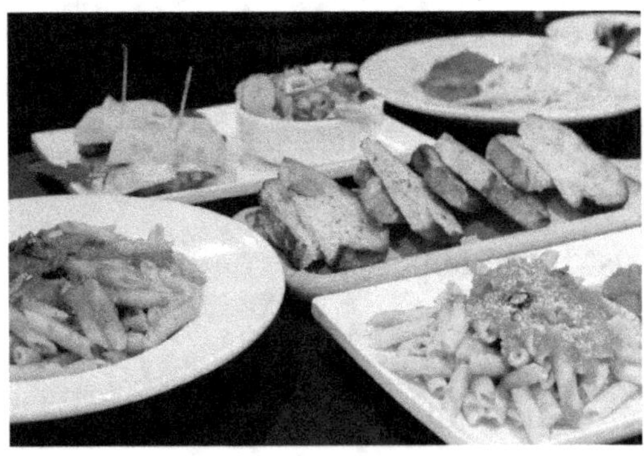

Dinner

1. Quinoa with asparagus with grilled salmon

Overview: A wholesome supper rich in fibre and omega-3 fatty acids that includes grilled salmon, quinoa, and asparagus.

In all, thirty minutes
Servings: Two

Ingredients:
- A pair of salmon fillets
- One cup cooked quinoa
- 2 tablespoons of olive oil and one bunch of trimmed asparagus
- To serve, cut lemon wedges

- According to taste, add salt and pepper.

Directions:

1.Set the oven or grill to preheat.

2. Salt and pepper are used to season fish. 3. 3. After cooking through, grill or bake.

4. Add salt, pepper, and olive oil to the asparagus. Preheat the grill or roast till soft.

5. Alongside grilled asparagus, place fish over quinoa. Lemon wedges are used as a garnish.

Nutritional Information

One hundred fifty calories

Protein: thirty grams

20 grams of good fats

Fibre: 8 g

2. Bell Peppers Stuffed with Vegetables

Overview: These stuffed bell peppers are a fantastic plant-based meal that are packed with veggies, black beans, and quinoa. They provide a filling and high-fibre meal.

45 minutes total time
Four servings

Ingredients:
- Quartered and seeded four bell peppers
- One cup cooked quinoa
- Rinse and drain one can of black beans
- 1 cup of kernel corn
- 1 cup finely chopped cherry tomatoes
- 1/2 cup coarsely chopped red onion
- one tsp cumin
- One-tsp chilli powder
- The optional half cup of shredded cheese

• fresh cilantro for the garnish

Directions:

1.Set oven temperature to 375°F, or 190°C.

2. Toss the quinoa, black beans, corn, tomatoes, onion, cumin, and chilli powder in a bowl.

3. Place a filling of the quinoa mixture into each half of the pepper.

4. Transfer to a baking dish, then bake for half an hour, covered with foil.

5. Bake for a further ten minutes after uncovering, sprinkling with cheese, if preferred.

6. Add some fresh cilantro as a garnish before presenting.

Nutritional Information

350 calories.

Protein: fifteen grams

Fibre: ten grams

Calcium: 150 mg

3. stir-fried chicken and veggies

Overview: An easy and tasty supper choice that's high in nutrients is a stir-fry made with lean chicken, vibrant veggies, and a ginger-soy sauce.

25 minutes in total

Servings : 3

Ingredients:

- Thinly cut one-pound chicken breast
- Cucumber florets, two cups
- one sliced bell pepper
- One carrot, cut into ribbons
- A single cup of snap peas
- Two teaspoons of low-sodium soy sauce
- 1 tablespoon finely chopped ginger
- A tsp of sesame oil
- two tsp olive oil

Brown rice to be served.

Directions:

1.In a wok or pan, preheat the olive oil. 2.Cook the chicken until browned after adding it.

3 Add the carrot, snap peas, bell pepper, and broccoli. Vegetables should be stir-fried until they are crisp-tender.

4. Stir together the sesame oil, ginger, and soy sauce in a small basin. Dollop the veggies and chicken on top.

5. Mix well until thoroughly cooked and coated.

6. On top of brown rice, serve.

Nutritional Information

400 calories.

Protein: 25 grams

12 grams of good fats

Fibre: 8 g

4. Avocado and Quinoa in a Black Bean Bowl

Overview: This nutritious and stomach-friendly supper choice is a protein-rich bowl with quinoa, black beans, avocado, and a zesty lime vinaigrette.

In all, thirty minutes
Servings: Two

Ingredients:
- One can of black beans
- one cup cooked quinoa
- one avocado
- one halved red onion
- one drained and rinsed can of beans
- two tablespoons fresh cilantro
- one chopped lime

- two teaspoons olive oil, and one teaspoon chopped red onion
- According to taste, add salt and pepper.

Directions:

1.Add the avocado, cherry tomatoes, red onion, cilantro, black beans, and quinoa to a bowl.

2. Combine the olive oil, lime juice, salt, and pepper in a small bowl.

3. Mix the quinoa mixture with the dressing after pouring it over it.

4. Utilise bowls for serving.

Nutritional Information

There are 420 calories.

Protein: fifteen grams

20 grams of good fats

Fibre: 12 grams

5. Curry made with veggies and lentils

Overview: An excellent plant-based supper choice is this delicious curry made with lentils, veggies, and spices.

Forty minutes in total.
Four servings

Ingredients:
- One cup of dried lentils, one washed onion, one diced bell pepper, one chopped, two sliced potatoes, two carrots, and one can coconut milk
- curry powder in two teaspoons
- One teaspoon of turmeric
- one tsp cumin
- According to taste, add salt and pepper.
- fresh cilantro for the garnish
- Basmati rice to be served.

Directions:

1.Lentils, veggies, curry powder, cumin, turmeric, and salt and pepper should all be combined in a saucepan.

2. Simmer until the lentils and veggies are cooked, about 25 to 30 minutes after bringing to a boil.

3. Top with freshly chopped cilantro and serve over basmati rice.

Nutritional Information

Total calories: 380

18g of protein.

15g of healthy fats

Fibre content: 14g

6. Stuffed Chicken Breast with Feta and Spinach

Overview: Dinner was a delicious dish of chicken breasts packed with feta and spinach, which provided protein and vital elements for intestinal health.

35 minutes in total.
Servings: Two

Ingredients:

- Boneless and skinless two chicken breasts
- Half a cup of crumbled feta cheese and two cups of fresh spinach
- two minced cloves of garlic
- a single spoonful of olive oil
- One-tsp dried oregano
- According to taste, add salt and pepper.
- To serve, cut lemon wedges

Directions:

1.Set oven temperature to 200°C, or 400°F.

2. Melt the garlic, add the olive oil, and sauté the spinach until it wilts.

3. Split a pocket in each breast of chicken and fill it with feta and sautéed spinach.

4. Add salt, pepper, and oregano for seasoning.

5. When the chicken is thoroughly cooked, bake it for 25 to 30 minutes.

6. Garnish with wedges of lemon.

Nutritional Information

Total calories: 380

Protein: forty grams

15g of healthy fats

5 grams of fibre

7. Skewers with shrimp and veggies

Overview: These shrimp and vegetable skewers are grilled to perfection, providing a low-calorie, high-protein supper option that is pleasant and light.

Twenty minutes overall
Servings : 3

Ingredients:

- Peeled and deveined one pound of shrimp
- one sliced zucchini
- 1 bell pepper, sliced into pieces
- Sliced into wedges, one red onion
- two tsp olive oil
- One tsp lemon juice
- One-teaspoon paprika with smoke
- According to taste, add salt and pepper.

Directions:

1 .Grill pan or grill at a high heat.

2. Add olive oil, lemon juice, smoked paprika, salt, and pepper to a bowl and toss to combine shrimp, zucchini, bell pepper, and red onion.

3. skewers with thread.

4 The vegetables should be soft and the shrimp opaque after grilling for 5 to 7 minutes, rotating them once.

5. Present at once.

Nutritious Information

300 calories.

Protein: 25 grams

15g of healthy fats

6 grams of fibre

To cap off your day with something tasty and nutritious, these dinner recipes not only put an emphasis on gut health but also provide a range of flavours and nutrients. Make necessary dietary adjustments and adjustments to the ingredients and portions based on personal tastes. Incorporate these filling and healthy dinners into a well-rounded, gut-friendly diet.

Conclusion:

Putting Your Gut Health First for a Happy and Meaningful Life

Let's review the main ideas from our investigation into the complex link between gut health and emotional well-being and urge you to prioritise gut health as the cornerstone of a happy and meaningful life as we draw to a close.

Synopsis of Main Ideas

Relevance of the Gut-Brain Axis:
Our gut and brain communicate dynamically via the gut-brain axis, which impacts our overall

health on both a physical and emotional level. Seeing this link emphasises how our emotions and mood are shaped by the state of our stomach.

The stomach is the primary site of serotonin production. Serotonin is a neurotransmitter that is essential for mood control. Sustaining a healthy gut environment is crucial for promoting the creation of serotonin, which in turn promotes emotional stability and a pleasant outlook.

Emotional Resilience and Gut Microbiota Diversity: Emotional resilience and gut microbiota diversity are related. An abundant and varied microbiome promotes a more robust gut-brain axis, which in turn elevates mood and lowers the likelihood of mood disorders.

Mood Impact of Inflammation: Mood problems are linked to chronic inflammation in the gut. Proactively supporting emotional well-being may be achieved by controlling inflammation via lifestyle decisions, such as nutrition and stress reduction.

Stress and Gut Health Interaction: There is a reciprocal association between stress and gut health. An unbalanced gut may lead to elevated stress levels, and chronic stress can upset the equilibrium of the gut microbiota. The development of a healthy gut environment requires the use of stress management techniques.

Actionable steps toward a happy and fulfilling life include adopting mindful eating, consuming probiotics and prebiotics, getting regular exercise, emphasising restful sleep, spending time in nature, practising mindfulness meditation, building strong relationships, expressing gratitude, and indulging in enjoyable activities.

Motivating Gut Health as a Priority

It's easy to forget how much of an influence gut health may have on our mental wellbeing in the daily grind. The following advice to put your gut health first should be kept in mind as we negotiate the challenges of contemporary living:

- **Holistic well-being:** Understand that physical, mental, and emotional components all contribute to well-being, which is a holistic term. Making gut health a priority is a crucial first step in living a healthy, balanced life.

- **Acceptance of the Mind-Body Connection:** Recognize that our emotional moods are greatly influenced by the food we put into our bodies. Emotional balance is facilitated by a healthy gut that has a good knock-on impact.

- **Empowerment via Decision-Making**: Recognize that you have influence over a lot of factors of your gut health. Your gut health and emotional resilience are directly impacted by every decision you make, ranging from what you eat to the lifestyle choices you make.

Investing in your total well-being over the long run is what makes prioritising gut health rather than just a passing fad. Knowing that these decisions contribute to a lifetime of happiness, vigour, and contentment, cultivate behaviours that promote a healthy gut flora.

- **Professional Advice**: You should think about seeing a healthcare provider, a nutritionist, or a holistic practitioner if you feel overwhelmed by the complexity of gut health. With their experience, they may provide specialised advice and methods made to fit your particular requirements.

In summary, the path back to experiencing pleasure in every moment is closely linked to your gut health. Keep in mind that little adjustments made consistently might result in big improvements as you set out on your journey. Make your digestive system a priority, adopt happy living techniques, and see the transformation of your emotional terrain. Cheers to a joyful, fulfilled life and the lively well-being that comes from a stomach that is in good health!